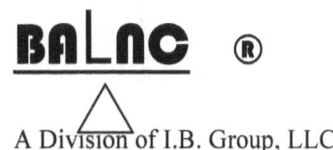

A Division of I.B. Group, LLC

Presents

"Improving Balance, Improving Lives"

By

Barb Paschal

(Physical Therapist, retired)

"Improving Balance, Improving Lives"

The intellectual property of I. B. Group, LLC

Copyright 2008

Revised second edition **2015**

Disclaimer

Chapter One:

"Fundamentals of Balance"

In this chapter you will:
- Be introduced to six Basic Balance Elements
- Learn how to Decrease Your Vulnerability to Falling
- Discover Three Ways to Improve Balance
- Examine the Complex Components of Balance

Basic Balance Elements

1) **Balance can be improved at any age** and despite most pre-existing conditions. How much you can improve is dependent on:

    A) Your awareness of how well you are practicing the **components of balance,** including frequent self-evaluation and correction.

    B) The type and extent of your pre-existing conditions.

2) **Balance is a very complex capacity**. Your balance is dependent upon many different parts of both your brain and your body. These parts interact with one another by exchanging information, to overcome "imbalance" (i.e. falling or unsteadiness) and to achieve "balance" (i.e. stability or control in motion or at rest). How quickly your body exchanges this brain-body information is called

"response timing", and it is a critical factor in your capacity for balance.

3) Our bodies and brains are born to continually seek balance. Injuries, diseases, birth defects, and genetic markers can alter your balance. The extent of that alteration, in most cases, can be overcome to varying degrees. **The brain can relearn** to accommodate to most pre-existing, or acquired conditions and increase your ability to balance. The severity of these conditions can vary, and as such, may require you to work harder to achieve an improvement in your balance. Improving balance is a natural capacity and many people have improved their balance and their lives with determination and diligence. The good news is the choice is yours; you can learn to improve your balance.

4) **Balance does decrease somewhat with age**; however research has not pinpointed a singular cause for this diminishment. This may be because of the complexity of balance and the body's ability for accommodation. Most retirees become relatively inactive in their retirement out of choice before necessity. In retirement days are often filled with quieter hobbies and pastimes, and with less emphasis on "physical activities". This diminishment of physical activity may play a much greater roll in the decrease in balance than age.

5) **Balance is a dynamic skill;** therefore, to significantly improve balance, it must be practiced while you are moving. Trying to improve balance by standing temporarily on one leg, (a form of static balance training) will not significantly improve your balance. Worse yet,

many who have tried to improve their balance through this static technique have gained little, and have stopped trying, with the misbelief that they can't improve. You can improve your balance and you can reteach your brain to accommodate to most pre-existing conditions, even recent inactivity. Your time and energy are precious; make the most of those resources by practicing balance while moving. By doing so, you greatly increase the level of reflex / response timing, and the other twelve components of balance, and thereby giving your brain a better chance to regain its/your capacity for balance.

6) **Like any skill, balance must be practiced**. Practice balance in all ways every day; make it a part of your life. Later you will learn how to make "well practiced balance" part of your daily living. For now, it is enough that you recognize that the more integrated in thought and action balance is in your pattern of living; the better balance you will achieve. Doing balance exercises two or three times a week, while not incorporating balance into daily living, is not the path to success. Live your life in **Better Balance** by being aware all day of how you move and move more often.

Decreasing your Vulnerability to Falling

Eighty percent of falls occur in the home. As startling as this finding is; it is true. It is primarily true for two reasons: first, you are most relaxed in your home and therefore your choices regarding balance tend to become your good or bad balance habits: secondly, you spend a great deal of time in your home. Most of your balance practice, good or bad, goes on in your home. Scene of the crime or classroom the choice is yours. As odd as it sounds you are both teacher and student when it comes to developing your habits. Therefore it is essential that you practice good balance habits at home. You already have a front row seat in the classroom, so let's focus on learning.

Fear of Falling is natural in all of us. Sometimes, however, this fear overwhelms our good judgment and leads to poor choices. Although we believe that the choices we make and habits we develop are meant to keep us from falling, they can in certain circumstances, actually make us more vulnerable to falling.

The following examines **four common issues associated with fear of falling**. In each there exists a wide range of possibilities from "I never do that" to "I always do that" and everywhere in between. Likewise a range exists from "I must do that" to "I do that, but I don't think I have to". It is impossible here to evaluate your personal circumstance, and as such, tell you what you specifically should or should not do regarding each of these issues. The intent is to provide you with an understanding of each issue so that you will be better informed about how these issues relate to falling. **Before deciding on any plan of action you should consult your Health Care Provider.**

1) **Reaching out** to walls and furniture as people move throughout their homes causes them to walk in postures that make them more vulnerable to falling. Although they do this believing that it makes them more secure it may be doing quite the opposite. If the brain is repetitively given the signal that bending, reaching, and using furniture to help support the body's weight, then it will learn to accommodate. At the same time it learns that the need for normal posture and balance are no longer needed. As such people are robbed of their future ability to balance correctly, and their muscle strength is diminished. They are now more at risk of falling because, if the wall isn't there, or the furniture slips, their weakened sense of balance and diminished strength will fail to stabilize them.

On the other hand, if people truly need assistance with balance, they need to consult with their doctor and get appropriate medical equipment. Canes, and walkers, etc. can help people, **who use them properly.** They may help you have good posture, and improve balance if they are the proper height and used correctly. It's a fact, people who constantly reach out to walls and furniture as they move throughout their home are at risk of falling. Therefore use a cane or a walker if you need to touch something to help you balance

2) **Shuffling or scuffing the feet will cause people to fall**. Shuffling and scuffing causes a poor walking pattern and leads to the eventual weakening of all the muscles in the legs. People who scuff or shuffle their feet usually fall

because they catch their toe on the edge of something. When that happens they lack the ability to recover quickly enough to avoid the fall. The inability to react quickly is a combination of, as previously discussed, reflex-response timing and muscle strength. Scuffing or shuffling greatly slows the reaction time in a person's ankle and toe muscles. These muscles are intended to lift the toes and ankles up when stepping forward, allowing the heel of the foot to land first. What starts as a bad habit choice, can eventually become a loss of ability. The good news is that by choosing the new good habit of toes up, stride forward, and heel landing first; strength, response timing, and thereby balance can improve.

3) Bending forward as you walk can cause a fall. We are meant to stand and walk in postural alignment; Head over neck, neck over shoulders, shoulders over hips, legs, and feet. Doing so sends the correct type of signals to our brains, strengthens our muscles, and maintains our reflex-response timing. Bending forward forces your body out of position. It bends your neck, back, hips, and knees, and causes you to redistribute, in a forward direction, the weight you place on your feet. You need each of these parts of your body performing at its best, standing ready to help should a sudden situation like a stumble or misstep occur. However by bending forward while you move forward, you have your body out of alignment, and in a position of poor advantage at a time of vulnerability. You may think bending forward is a defensive strategy against falling. The truth is quite the opposite; it can actually be part of the cause for the fall. Practice standing and walking in as good a posture as you can, you will become an ally in improving balance.

4) Moving or walking slowly, at a rate or level below what we are really capable of, when combined with poor posture can contribute to potential falls. The words slowly and briskly are relative terms, and have a different meaning for each of us based on our sense of being safe. We must give some thought to our individual circumstance, weighing where we are against the goal of where we want to be. The focus here is moving more briskly, but only incrementally increasing the rate of movement commensurate with your specific circumstance and safety.

Most of us have a natural walking ability. When we specifically focus on our walking, many of us walk a little more briskly and carry ourselves in better postural alignment; we stand more upright more closely approximating our natural ability. Our postural alignment, the natural coordination of head, neck, back, legs, and arm swing are critical to balance. Our brains are pre-programmed to this coordinated combination of movements. Practicing moving more briskly and concentrating on posture improves your balance and strengthens the very muscles needed for better balance. Moving more slowly and without concentrating on the postural alignment of the body, we tend to be slightly, even sometimes significantly, off balance. Subsequently we are less likely to keep our balance and therefore more likely to fall.

Ways to Improve Balance

Nearly everyone can improve their balance somewhat. Some of those who could improve lack the determination to try, and some lack the diligence to persist in the attempt. But for those who believe they can improve and persevere in that belief; those stalwarts want and deserve a clear, concise, and common sense way forward.

1) Improve your postural alignment. Head over neck, neck over shoulders, shoulders over hips, legs, and feet; you need to stand and move upright. Realign your core alignment again and again all day long. Make it a habit. This effort is especially important in your home, since you spend the major portion of every day there. The payoff for this labor will be banked in your brain, as a good balance habit. As an added bonus doing it will get easier over time because you will be building both muscle strength and endurance. Postural alignment is perhaps the single most important issue you can address; and doing so gets easier sooner than you might think.

Everyone can improve their postural or core alignment at least somewhat; and every bit helps. If you have a permanent deformity in your spine that doesn't allow you to stand as straight as you used to; do what you can. Make it your best effort. We all tend to "slouch". This happens many times each and every day. Just because it is typical of all of us doesn't make it acceptable. If you make a concerted effort to work on it, your ability to sit, stand, and move correctly will become the norm, rather than the exception. Each of us could stand and sit at least a little straighter. Make your best effort to check and correct your core alignment often.

Imagine you have a line from your ears to your ankles like a side-seam. Now think about your shoulders in relation to your side-seam. Your shoulders should be on, not forward nor behind, that imaginary line from ear to ankle. Here's a surprise; the palms of your hands will tell you if your shoulders are on that line, your side-seam. Check now to see where your palms naturally rest when you stand; stand as you would have before you started reading this book. If your palms are forward, and closer to the front of your thigh, your shoulders are forward of the line also. If your palms are closer to the back of your thigh, your shoulders are behind the line. Now you can tell, anywhere and anytime, whether you're "slouching" (palms forward=shoulders too far forward), or "over achieving" (palms back=shoulders too far back).

Most people "slouch". If you are "slouching", you are probably standing with your head forward, your chin forward, and your shoulders rolled forward. To correct "slouching" do the following three things in order. First, imagine that your head is being pulled up and slightly back by a string attached to its top; go ahead and be pulled gently up and slightly back. Second, pull your chin in and slightly downward, but again, be gentle. Third, pull your shoulder blades closer to your spine and downward a little toward your waist until your palms hang naturally along your side-seam. It is important that your palms arrive at your side-seam because of these three steps, and not because you simply moved them to that position.

Fewer people are "overachievers". If you are "overachieving", you are most likely arching your back or leaning a bit backward from the waist. To correct "leaning back from the waist" or "arching" don't bother rolling your shoulders forward; that probably won't help you as much as you might think. Instead, you can bring your shoulders closer to your side-seam by concentrating on gently pulling your shoulder blades closer to your spine, and downward a little bit toward your waist. At the same time, if you have been leaning backward from the waist make a conscious effort to straighten, by bending forward ever so slightly at the waist. Note, bending your neck isn't what's needed here. Having done these two postural realignments, your palms should hang naturally along that imaginary line from your ear to your ankle.

In either case, realigning your posture involves small, but focused movements. Self-evaluate your alignment and ask yourself: where is/are my head, shoulders, neck, back, hips, and feet? Do this self-evaluation often during each day, and then make your adjustments, as described above. These small increments of movement with repetition over time will become your natural and everyday posture. It may feel awkward at first. If practiced consistently, however, you will feel not only more comfortable, but it may also alleviate a good deal of neck, back and shoulder stiffness. Remember, you were born with the natural ability to stand and move in excellent postural alignment. As a child, you were active and moved in good alignment. Your brain will recognize you sitting, standing and moving in alignment again. It will relearn and retain the lessons of good postural habits.

2) Improve your Body Mechanics. This section is intended to introduce you to the concept of body mechanics, which is effectively "postural alignment in motion".

You can find much more on this subject in **Chapter Two.**

Body mechanics is moving your body in correct alignment, in everything you do throughout your day. Activities such as: reaching to a shelf, pulling a rake, pushing a wheelbarrow, lifting a box, putting a heavy pot on the stove, moving a casserole from the oven to the counter, digging a hole, gardening, shoveling snow, getting up or down from a chair, on or off the toilet, in or out of the car, playing with a grandchild, mopping the floor, vacuuming, getting groceries, or getting out of the car. Using good postural alignment in everyday tasks can help strengthen your muscles and improve your balance. Or, in the absence of good alignment, your daily activities can be prime contributors to injuries and falls. Good alignment builds strength and balance; poor alignment allows important muscles to weaken and makes you more vulnerable to falling. It's an easy choice, and it's your to make.

3) Exercise can improve your balance. Exercise is Key to Balance. Your understanding of how and why exercise is fundamental to improving your balance.

Previously, we discussed the inter-connection of your brain and your body. When the body moves, it moves in a specific way. Your brain sends signals to various parts of your body, determined by the specific movement you desire. Your brain also receives signals from the body's specific movement that tells the brain how that movement was made. The brain and body interact in this manner both teaching and learning at the same time. If, through your conscious effort of thought, your brain tells your body to move in good postural alignment and in accordance with your current strength and coordination; you're off to a good start. Now, if you do it often enough, your brain will recognize a repetitive pattern. It will remember that this is precisely how this specific movement is to be done. With enough repetition, you will have taught your brain a good balance lesson, created a good balance habit, and improved your strength, and coordination for that movement. All of these pieces add up to a new definition of your improved balance.

But that's not all. The very act of repetition improves your "response timing". When you think of "response", picture a muscle-brain two way conversation. For "timing", picture a rapid, brain-nerve-muscle three way conversation, on this new pathway. In this illustrative and conceptual realm of "response timing", movements made in good postural alignment ultimately leads to good brain lessons learned. If repeated consistently, a new good habit will develop, which is your goal. Remember that although this explanation is simplified to illustrate the concept, there are many complex parts of your brain and an intricate network of interactions with your muscles and nerves that, under proper conditions, can improve your balance. An added benefit to improved balance is the improvement of both your muscle strength, and how quickly that strength comes into play when you need it to catch yourself.

However, if you practice movements in poor alignment the process we just examined still operates; but it will result in a bad lesson. It will lead to a bad habit; and it also makes you more vulnerable to falls.

Therefore, you need to do it properly; and you need to do it repetitively. What does that look like? First, what that doesn't look like is a schedule of exercises only done 20 times in a row, 3 days a week. What it does look like is your everyday activity. What everyday activity looks like is just that; what you do all day long. Use the energy you are going to use anyway, but use your energy to its best outcome. You have limited energy and time. Don't waste precious moments of opportunity during your day. By integrating good habits into everyday activities you can expect to improve your balance, strength, flexibility, and safety. The important addition is that you're making a concerted effort to live your life in good postural alignment. You will be helping to buy back some of the ability to balance that has been slipping away for years. Walking, sitting down in, or rising up from your favorite chair, standing, cleaning, cooking, and gardening all the things that make up your day become your exercise. It is exercise that you are constantly living. Quickly, you won't even think of it as exercise anymore. You'll be doing more and enjoying your health more; because you chose to improve your balance and as a result, improved your life.

One last thought, in addition to the above, you should do or work up to doing thirty minutes of aerobic exercise everyday. Walking, swimming, bicycling and aerobic exercise classes are examples of aerobic activity. By doing so, you will improve your strength, endurance, flexibility, and overall health. Understand however, that you must give due thought to your specific health and circumstance. **Ask your Health Care Provider for advice before you begin an aerobic exercise program or significantly increase one you already have.**

Complex Components of Balance

Balance is very complex. What we know as balance involves at least twenty different parts of the body and the brain. In this section we will discuss some of these parts and their interactions.

The first three of these: Vision, Hearing, and Vestibular System, can be improved only **with the help of your Health Care Provider**.
Very briefly:
1) Vision: visual inputs to your brain help you balance by orienting you spatially; your orientation to the horizon.
2) Hearing: auditory cues help you balance by orienting you to those things that share your surroundings; cars, rain, wind, people, cats, etc.
3) Vestibular System: helps you balance by providing sensory input to your brain about the motion of your body.

You are experiencing some degree of concern regarding your balance. It is an important first step, to attend to the three components above by **consulting with your Health Care Provider.** Through this consultation, you'll establish the best possible foundation for moving forward. Skip this important step and you seriously reduce the effectiveness and end product of your precious effort and could, depending on your specific circumstance, put you at risk. It's your choice; make the right choice.

The rest of what will be covered in this section is the components that you can work to improve.

4) Postural Alignment is perhaps the most important component in this group. Chapter two is primarily focused on this component, and will serve as your guide to understanding the key role it plays in your balance throughout your day.

5) Muscle Strength provides the mechanical power to sustain balance while stationary, or more importantly, while in motion. Muscles are strengthened or built through use. If they are not used they weaken or atrophy. If the key to muscle strength is use, then how they are used is an important factor in how quickly they develop and to what degree that development takes place. Each part of your body, from your feet all the way up to your head, plays a role. By standing up as straight as you can, in good postural alignment, you place your muscles in the best position to gain strength from your effort. But only by moving in that posture, as you go about your everyday activities, will you develop the strength that you need and desire. Postural alignment gives you potential, but when you add the motion of everyday activities, you'll turn that potential into the product you want, increased muscle strength. As your strength increases, your activities become easier because your balance will have improved.

6) Joint Flexibility is a major factor in determining your capacity for movement. Your ability to move is needed to keep your muscles as limber as possible. This in turn allows you to achieve good postural alignment, hence better balance.

Prevention is the first thing upon which you should focus. The best rule of thumb is to try limiting your sitting to less than thirty minutes at any one time. After thirty minutes, get up and move. More movement is better, but if you only walk to another room and back; it's better than having not walked at all. This periodic movement will help your back, hips, knees, ankles, and feet from tightening up. Conversely, if you sit and don't move periodically, you can expect that the muscles in these body parts will tighten, your flexibility will be diminished, your posture will degrade, and your balance will be impaired. You undoubtedly have had this experience, at times, after sitting for just an hour. Getting up and moving around, in certain situations, is sometimes easier said than done. Driving or being in a theater is an example. In these situations try this: straighten your knees, pull your toes up toward your shins, and make circles with your ankles. Remember more movement is better, but any is better than none.

Keeping your body in good postural alignment will assist you in slowing muscle tightening. If you are sitting make sure your lower back, your lumbar region, is supported. You can do this by placing a pillow between your low back and the chair or the couch. By providing your back this needed support, you also help place your hips, shoulders, and neck in good alignment so they are less likely to tighten as you sit. When you get up you'll be less tight, more flexible, and will therefore move in better balance.

Don't shuffle or scuff your feet! If you shuffle, you decrease the muscles' movement and decrease strength. This in turn reduces your ability to move, negatively affects your pattern of movement, and ultimately reduces the flexibility of your joints. As a result, your balance is impaired and you are more vulnerable to falling. If you've been shuffling, start work on improving your walking pattern in small but increasing increments. Although like anything that you haven't practiced in a while, it may feel odd, or even difficult. With a conscious and concerted effort you can improve.

Gently swing your arms as you walk. Swinging your arms at your sides in a natural fashion anytime you walk can help to keep your shoulders and back flexible. In addition, try moving them out to the side and overhead frequently during your day. You already know it by now; more movement equates to more flexibility!

Stretching is important, however specific stretching exercises for each joint, while they exist, are beyond the scope of this book. Each joint can benefit from stretching, but **your specific needs regarding stretching require the professional evaluation of your Health Care Provider.** Each person's individual case is different, and requires personal evaluation. Visiting your Health Care Provider may result in valuable information specific to your individual needs. Daily stretching is important to joint flexibility, movement, and balance. You'll feel better, be more in control, have better balance, and be safer in the bargain. Look into it; you'll be glad you did.

7) Endurance, without it your balance and safety are at risk. Endurance is the ability to sustain active physical activity over time. Often our estimate of endurance, our sense of lethargy or peppiness, is subjective. That estimate can vary significantly from an objective measurement of endurance.

Your body stores energy and it also uses energy. Endurance is the measure of your body's ability to turn stored energy into your physical activity. This ability can change; and the good news is your endurance can gradually increase through increasing your exercise time: don't guess, look at your watch. **If possible, slowly increase the length of time you exercise before you increase the level of difficulty.** This is safer for your body, and especially your joints.

Your muscles need energy to work; and the work they do is generally thought of as strength. Previously, you learned that strength is directly proportional to your ability to balance. Within reason more strength usually means better balance. Your endurance is the measure of the energy your muscles can draw upon to run your body over a period of time. Your endurance also depends on your cardio-pulmonary strength. Your heart is a muscle, and there are muscles in the bronchial walls in your lungs. These muscles only maintain and build their strength through endurance exercise. Building your endurance requires doing more physical activity over a longer period of time. For example, walking five minutes at a time builds a little endurance, but walking twenty minutes at a time builds more. If you have some endurance now, you can expect to have more if you become more physically active. You will lose what you've gained however, if you don't maintain an increased level of activity. Remember exercise builds endurance and strength which are two of the major components of the physical foundation of balance.

Wow! So exercise is the good news! Do you have a specific exercise program: walking, swimming, or bicycling? If you don't, you may want to consider starting one, but before you do, **talk with your Health Care Provider before you begin an exercise program**.

If you have a program, you can build your endurance by incrementally extending your workouts. If you walk outside or on your treadmill 15-20 minutes a day, three times a week, consider adding a day to your week. After you become comfortable with the initial change, add another day, and so on. If you do aerobics 2-3 times a week, consider adding another session to your week; put on the music and do it in your home. Or you could supplement your aerobics by adding walking to your program. As you increase your routine exercise, you will increase your endurance. Depending on your current level of fitness, your initial efforts will be rewarded with an observable increase in endurance. This will provide you with more energy for your everyday activities, as well as your exercise program. You'll know this is happening because your usual workout will seem easier, or more comfortable. Each time your program becomes comfortable, you might want to consider increasing it further. You will make your own judgment, but an optimal exercise session includes 5-10 minutes of warm-up exercises, 30+ minutes of moderate aerobic exercises, 5-10 minutes of cool-down exercises, and 5-10 minutes of stretching exercises.

An optimal program would make exercise part of every day, seven days a week. To be at its best your body needs daily exercise. Hopefully you've noticed that daily activities are good, but they are not a substitute for exercise. Sitting, reading, or watching TV, aren't exercise; a walk with the dog is a bit better, but considering the slow pace and frequent stops it isn't exercise that will build endurance. Don't be misled by articles purporting that raking leaves, gardening, or parking further from a store's front door are a substitute for enough exercise to make enough difference in your balance.

An exercise program is important. If you don't have one, talk to your Health Care Provider, and ask their advice about starting an exercise program appropriate for you. If you already have one; consider expanding it. Endurance builds in proportion to exercise up to a reasonable limit. Endurance and strength, built through exercise, along with the balance lessons previously covered, are some of the safeguards against falls. You'll have increased your ability to catch yourself, and in a way turned your exercise into your safety net.

8) Sensation is the "feeling" your sensory system provides. Your sensory system needs frequent input to give you the best feedback. When you move your body multiple times a day in many directions, (forward, backward, and to the side, etc.), your brain receives many sensory messages from various parts of your body. New research has shown that, given an increase in the amount of input, your brain is capable of increasing the number of synapses; the nerve-brain connections called neurological pathways you have in your brain. This improves your brain's capacity to recognize the need for and respond with better balance. The more you move correctly, the more the input from that movement reinforces these new pathways. Your good lessons over time can reteach your brain to better respond to your balance needs.

9) You have multiple "Higher Centers" of your brain. There are centers in the cerebellum and the cerebrum that help you control movement, memory, intention, logic, learning, responses to sensory input, as well as visual, and auditory inputs. You might call these higher centers the "Grand Central Station" in your brain. They help you understand what to practice to improve your balance, why and how to practice it, and tell you how well you are doing in practicing your balance lessons. Your continuous and concerted effort to apply what we've been discussing as good balance lessons is important.

10)   Safety Awareness is always thinking ahead. Because eighty percent of falls occur in the home, you become the "safety awareness officer in charge". Your next fall is most likely to happen in your home, absent your effort. Do your duty; look around and change, remove, or remedy as many obstacles to your balance as you can. Here's a short list to get you started:

"Sloppy Slippers" make you shuffle, in order to keep these rascals on your feet. They tend to be loose fitting, backless and have little support. That soft comfy feeling belies the contribution they can make to the chances of your falling. You need support from your footwear in and out of the house. Every step you take, every foot fall should provide you the best possible foot placement. Good support will help place your feet, ankles, legs, hips, and back, in proper postural alignment. Buy a good pair of "inside shoes" and put them on when you come in the house.

Pick up throw rugs, and move electrical cords, purse straps, and foot stools, etc. Things trip you, and while you can't manage without them, make it your job to keep them out of the way.

Buy more automatic night lights. Put them in areas or passageways throughout your home. When the lights aren't on, you can't afford to be in the dark.

If you use a cane or a walker consult with a Physical Therapist, and ask them to adjust it to correctly match your needs. At least half of those using one or the other suffer from having them too short. Remember, bending forward takes you out of postural alignment and makes you more vulnerable to falls.

Check the condition of the rubber tips on your cane or walker, if you use one. Their purpose is to prevent the device from slipping suddenly and contributing to a fall. Check them routinely. As they wear out they require periodic replacement.

Keep your eyeglasses and hearing aids up to date. Proper hearing and vision are important to your balance. Been a while since you've had them checked? Now is the time to get an appointment.

11) Response Timing is a subject covered previously. By way of review, the more often you move in postural alignment, particularly in your everyday activities, the quicker your response time will become. This could mean the difference between catching yourself and falling. Strengthen your safety net; practice moving in good postural alignment at all times.

Chapter Two:

"Postural Alignment and Body Mechanics"

In this chapter you will:
- Learn ways to improve your balance immediately

Postural Alignment and Body Mechanics, while doing normal daily activities, are two of the three quickest ways to decrease your vulnerability to falls; the third being Exercise.

The new term for posture is "core alignment". It is a very accurate and often more helpful way of expressing what posture is all about. When we were growing up, we were often told to "stand up straight, shoulders back, stomach in, and chin in". We might do all those things for a few seconds; and we usually did them incorrectly. As such, we held our body tense, our shoulders too far back, held our breath to make our stomachs flatten, and our heads tipped backwards. Then we would drop back into a slump.

You need to find your best alignment, despite permanent deformities you may have. It's not hard, and it soon will begin to feel comfortable. Good alignment is where you were born to be. Until it becomes your natural habit, you'll need to reposition your body in your best postural alignment many times an hour. You need to do this whether you're sitting, standing, walking, or doing some other activity or task. Do not be discouraged to find yourself bending out of alignment; it's just another opportunity to realign to your best posture. It's normal to find yourself slipping at first; just keep trying. After all, if correcting old bad habits was a snap, you wouldn't be reading this.

Our world is "down". Counters are low, gardens are at our feet, tables are below, and children are small. We get so used to bending that we forget that we can be in good alignment and bend also. Bend your knees and hips instead of your spine. Postural/Core alignment is keeping the "core" of you, your head, spine, and pelvis well balanced on top of one another. Your pelvis contains the "sacrum" which is five vertebrae fused together to form part of your spine. Your pelvis also contains your hip sockets. Your shoulder blades contain the shoulder sockets and are connected to your spine via muscles and ligaments. Therefore, your core controls your entire body. If your core is in good alignment you can use your arms and legs to their best advantage, keeping them and you safe from injury. In addition, **poor alignment wears away at every joint in your body.**

By age seven or eight we have usually achieved great core alignment. This is due to all the running, jumping, climbing, etc. that develops balance in childhood. Later in the teen and adult years we often lose some of our good body "sense". The effect is that we begin to stand, walk and generally move in less than great alignment. In part this is attributable first to teenage self-conscious postures and then the busy days of adulthood filled with family, job, house and yard. It takes our mind off our own health. Time flies by and we finally reach retirement. We find ourselves slowing down and taking time to relax. We become immersed in hobbies, volunteering, family and friends. We allow ourselves to believe that doing less physical activity is what retirement is all about. About this time we start noticing that we can't get out of chairs as easily anymore. Typically we chalk it all up to advancing age or arthritis instead of the fact that we have begun to sit longer and recognizing that through decreased activity we allowed our muscles to weaken. We sit hunched over hobbies, books, computers, watching TV and then think we can't straighten up easily because of our age. We next to never think that the weakness and stiffness throughout our bodies is caused by our level of inactivity and that our postural/core alignment in those activities is a few points south of good. Consequently, we have to relearn the posture of our early youth; an underappreciated gift because it was given to us automatically and for free. Now we have to retrain our brains and bodies to sit, stand, walk, and do every day normal activities in good postural alignment and use good body mechanics. So, let's get started.

The good news is that it is actually very possible for everyone reading this book to improve their alignment and their balance somewhat. How much you improve depends on your pre-existing conditions and your commitment to your health. It also depends on your understanding of how your body works. In this book I have tried very earnestly to clarify how and why your body works as it does in the category of your balance. But make no mistake; you'll have to commit yourself to work at it! You'll have to think about it constantly. You'll have to understand what to do, and why doing it correctly is so very important. My belief in this possibility, recognizing that it takes a commitment of effort, is why I write books, produce DVDs and lecture frequently on balance. I believe that if you will try, your balance will improve somewhat. Again, your pre-existing conditions to play a part in your potential for improvement. I've seen hundreds of people improve their balance at least somewhat and thereby improve their health and lives. If they can; you can. I want you to try; I want you to be able to live a better life, through better balance.

Core alignment is essential to everything we do. For instance, if you couldn't hold your spine in stable alignment and you were playing tennis or golf, the ball wouldn't go where you wanted it to go. Your limbs depend on your core stability in order to function properly. Stability depends on having a strong core musculature. That means that you must use your core as it was meant to be used and position it where it can do its best work. Your core musculature is made up of your spinal muscles and your abdominal muscles. There are literally hundreds of these muscles to help you. Remember there are many vertebrae that all connect together to make up your spine. As such, what you do with your neck directly affects your low back and vice versa. Core alignment isn't just putting you upright in proper alignment. It is also about holding you there as you move. Your abdominal muscles also help stabilize your core. The best way to strengthen them is to use them all day long in doing all your activities in core alignment.

Your spinal muscles are endurance muscles. Their cellular structure is capable of holding your whole spinal column in great posture for hours. If you can only hold your spine in good posture for a few seconds, then that's your starting point. Try holding your spine in good posture often during each day, and time how long you can hold it in that posture. The more you try this correctly; the sooner seconds will turn to minutes. In a few days you'll be able to hold better alignment, not only for a few minutes or more while sitting and standing, but also while walking. You'll have made a stride forward toward better balance.

When you lean forward it is more difficult for your body to maintain balance. Primarily, this is because your weight is being unevenly distributed. When your head, which weighs ten to twelve pounds, is forward on your neck, depending on the severity of the angle, leverage can cause its weight force to as much as triple. Here's an illustration; when you hold a heavy item near your body it's heavy; but if you try holding it out at arms length the same item will seem heavier. That's the effect of leverage. If you bend forward at your waist or hips, then at least half of your total body weight is out of alignment. If you weigh 120 pounds and bend forward to a cane, walker, or the furniture, you could be out of balance, in a forward manner, by up to 60 pounds. This puts undue stress on your hips, knees, ankles, and feet, as well as forcing you off balance. Your back muscles must now work harder to not let you bend even further forward, thus straining them, and causing pain and potential damage. The same sort of thing occurs if you lean to one side, lean backwards a bit, or stand with your weight unevenly distributed to one foot or the other. Too often, but not always, this happens for no other reason than it's a bad habit. Look in a full length mirror to evaluate your best posture, or ask a friend or family member to see if they can detect you being off center. Note, they can't help you evaluate, if you can't explain to them what good core alignment looks like! **If you need more help consult with your Health Care Provider.** A Physical Therapist can fully evaluate your alignment, help you know how to correct problems, and identify which muscles need strengthening.

The best way to strengthen your back muscles is to use them, as they were meant to be used, all day long. It does little good to do ten or twenty exercises at the gym and then "slump" the rest of the day. Always use prevention first. Don't slump in the chair or couch. Use a lumbar pillow, sit up as tall as you can, pull your chin in slightly, place your head over your neck, shoulders in the middle of that side seam, feet planted somewhat apart and flat on the floor; no leg crossing. You use your back muscles and abdominal muscles to their best advantage as you strive to sit in core alignment.

If you always lean back in a chair you waste potential chances to get stronger and thereby improve your balance. Remember spinal muscles are endurance muscles. Their reliable strength measured across time is how the endurance capacity is determined. Some strength, across a short time, may be your starting point, but good strength across more time is the path to follow. So take out your watch, sit up correctly, and measure your endurance. Write the result on your calendar. Practice at least ten times each day, measure again a week from now, and a month from now and see the improvement for yourself.

Some people believe their muscles relax while they slump. What's really true is that they weaken and stiffen in this poor position. When you sit upright and back in the chair with a lumbar pillow, your low back is actually more comfortable. Because this is more restful, you'll find you have more flexibility when, after no more than 30 minutes, you get to move around. Your body craves movement, alignment, and symmetry. It tells you when you've given it what it wants, and when it is deprived of the same. Flexibility is the reward message, and stiffness is the opposite message.

When you are on your feet, keep both feet a comfortable distance apart, distribute your weight evenly, and stand in great alignment. If you must carry something, carry it as symmetrically as you can. If you carry a purse, don't carry it in your hand, between elbow and ribs, or slung over your shoulder. Any of these make you asymmetrical, adversely affect your core alignment, can pull you off balance, interfere with you reflex-response, and may make you more vulnerable to falling. Use a small purse, with a strap that fits over your head and across one of your shoulders, crossing your body, front and back, diagonally. The purse stays in front for easy access, and both your arms and hands are free. You're symmetrical, and the added bonus is the purse is harder for some scoundrel to snatch away from you. You can take this tip to the bank!

Chapter Three

"Exercises Can Improve Your Balance"

In this chapter you will:
- Learn to walk with Precision and "Vigor"
- Turn getting in and out of a chair into a More Useful Purpose,
- Find the Magic in Music for you

Exercise is the third essential way to improve balance. Exercise can strengthen your muscles at any age. Which exercises each person needs are very specific and will not be covered in this book. Being evaluated by a Physical Therapist to find out which muscles need strengthening and stretching is incredibly helpful for your health. Your muscles will outlast your joints and protect them through strength. Protect your joints and your mobility by getting stronger. Let's see how easy getting stronger can be.

Let's start by discussing what I call **Walking with Precision and Vigor**. In your home you take many short walks, from room to room, throughout your day. You get something to drink, visit the bathroom, answer the phone, check the refrigerator, etc. Most of the time those moments of potential exercise are wasted; done with slow motions, taken with little concentration on either your postural alignment or how you place your feet.

You could have thought about each of those walks. You could have made them with as much vigor as you could muster. By having concentrated on walking with precision and planning, you could have moved closer to improving your strength and balance. More to the point, you could have done so without taking any extra time out of your busy day.

What is "vigor"? It is relative to what each of us can do; put simply, walk as briskly as you can. First, stand up as straight as you can. If you're stiff from sitting, the initial few seconds may not be as straight as those that follow. Keep working on your postural alignment through the entire walk. Swing your arms gently at your sides. Each arm swing strengthens your back. If you use a walker, of course you can't swing your arms, but the best thing for your back and balance is to make sure that you have been measured and that the walker is adjusted to fit you. Make sure you gently lift your toes and ankles as you begin your step and that your heel gently touches the floor first as you complete it. Stride out with as much joy and vitality as you can summon. If you have music playing, that will help as well, but more about music later.

Get up at least every thirty minutes, after the end of each chapter of your book, every other commercial, or after every second e-mail you write. Set a timer so that you don't get so immersed in your activity that you forget your health is calling you! If you volunteer somewhere; offer frequently to help with some task that requires you to get up and walk. Walking with precision and vigor, done many times a day can add numerous chances to cement balance practice into your daily activities, and thereby your mind and body. Most people comment that after trying this for a few days, that they hadn't realized how poorly they'd been walking and in such poor posture. By focusing on this new goal of walking with precision and vigor, they felt younger and more like they used to feel. Of course this plan is not restricted to inside your house. Apply it if you're on the treadmill or on a walk outside.

Remember to concentrate on what you're doing and how to get the most out of that effort. If you walk on a treadmill, try walking at a pace where you don't have to hold on to the bars on the front or side. If you need those bars, use them, but see if you can work up to just lightly touching the bars. As you strengthen and improve your balance; you may work up to not needing them as much or at all. Approach this as a goal; work at it, but be safe first. Do not bend over to read your book or watch the flashing numbers on the treadmill. Remember a correct postural alignment and proper walking pattern, toes and ankles up somewhat, heels down first, will absolutely change and improve your balance.

When you walk, don't put your hands in your pockets. If it's cold, put on some gloves or mittens. Swing your arms, they are part of your balance and they strengthen your back with each swing. When you walk with your hands in your pockets, it is almost impossible to stand as straight as you could otherwise. Walking a bit more briskly, with vigor, will make you use your side hip balancing muscles You will do better and you'll do less "wobble side-to-side" that slow walking encourages. Try this brisk walking in your home and concentrate on posture and precision. See if you can notice the difference it makes. If you do this frequently at least once every thirty minutes, or whenever you get up from your chair; you will steadily increase and reinforce a good balance lesson for your brain, as well as gain strength. Your brain will relearn that this is how you are to walk. Soon this exercise will have turned into a new habit. When you are ready, try this same brisk walking outside. It's exciting that you can choose to make opportunities that occur throughout your day exercises that will strengthen you, revitalize you, and make everyday a healthy day. Once you begin, you will hopefully take every opportunity to walk more often and in better ways. Although walkers, canes, splints, and braces may determine your pace, they do not have to keep you from this type of exercise.

Getting up and down from a chair, couch, or toilet is something you do many times a day. Why not make the most of it getting stronger and healthier in the bargain. Statistics show that many falls and injuries occur when you are getting in or out of a chair etc. The reasons:

1)Because of a lack of exercise your legs are weak.

2) By trying to get up from the back of the chair you disadvantage yourself by attempting to rise from a most difficult position; a difficult maneuver for even the most fit.

3) By rocking back and forth, using momentum to catapult you out of the chair, you don't build muscle strength and you risk throwing yourself off balance.

4) By holding your breath while you strain to get out of the chair, you run the risk of making yourself dizzy or worse fainting.

5) By twisting your back and pulling your knees and/or shoulders out of alignment, you risk pain and injury to your back that can cause you to fall.

6) By dropping into a chair you can actually break your tailbone.

This has become an issue for so many people, some as young as their 40's. Using this everyday activity as both a strengthening exercise and a way to keep you safer makes sense. The muscles called the quadriceps make up the entire front of your thighs. They are the main muscles that help you get up and down from the surfaces you sit upon. They are very large and tend to strengthen quickly. However, they also weaken quickly when not used accurately. Learn how to correctly and safely rise up from and lower yourself down to a chair from your Physical Therapist. Getting up or down slowly and carefully from a chair can safely strengthen your leg and core muscles. Each day you will build more strength, but if you stop you'll lose what you've worked so very hard for, quickly. So keep the thief at bay.

As with walking, getting up and down is a constant activity throughout your day. Now you can make it an exercise opportunity as well, but only if you do it correctly. **Precaution: if you need to use your arms, to help you up and down, as compensation for a lack of strength in your legs, do so. Across time you may progress to just a light touch or even no arms at all; you and your Therapist will be the judge.**

If you want to practice getting up and down from a chair, try not to do more than one or two in a row to begin with, so you don't make your muscles sore. More important than practicing in a row, is simply remembering to use these steps as you sit and rise throughout your day. You know that you're not supposed to sit more than thirty minutes before you get up and walk briskly; now you can add this to that exercise. You'll get stronger quicker, a "twofer"; what a deal!

If every chair in your house is a swivel, rocker, or very low then buy or borrow a good stable chair, i.e. a "straight" chair. After you get stronger your rockers, swivels and low chairs won't pose the same risk to your safety that they do today. The sooner you start to get up and down correctly the sooner your strength, control and balance will improve. You can improve to the point that any chair, couch, toilet or car seat that you encounter will be within your ability.

Music is a wonderful experience. Your brain is wired for music. Everyone's brain responds to music. It does not matter if you sing well or if you are able to read music or play a musical instrument. Research has found that music has a beneficial affect on many areas of the brain and subsequently a person's performance on a wide variety of tasks. Balance and memory and exercise are all tremendously and positively affected by music.

Exercise done correctly promotes strength, flexibility, endurance and reflex-response timing. As described in chapter one, you are re-teaching your brain. Music will improve what you gain from exercise. Surprise! You don't even have to play music; you can just sing or hum a song while you dance this exercise away.

Chapter Four

"Putting Your Best Foot Forward"

In this chapter you will:
- Come to understand the special importance of your feet and ankles.

Our feet and ankles play a special part in our Balance. Their strength comes primarily from muscles located in the lower leg: your calf and shin. The tendons from these muscles run across the ankles attaching to the top, bottom, and sides of the foot. The great number of sensory nerves, and special nerve signal centers in your feet and ankles are very important in helping you be less vulnerable to falling. They tell you: 1) details of the surface you are walking on such as the angles of rise and fall, front to back and side to side. 2) details of what you are doing with the rest of your body, such as leaning in a direction(s), or carrying enough of a load that your ankles and feet need to accommodate to it. Most of the time, we don't think about our feet. When we do, it's usually that we think of them as painful or problematic. However, the truth is that they are amazing. Stop and think of the millions of steps that they help us take in the course of our lives.

If you want the best use out of your ankles and feet, you have to move them often and well. Small steps, shuffling steps, or too few steps give only a small amount of input to these nerve and signal centers. You, therefore, only get a small amount of feedback from the nerve centers. You need all the input/feedback you can get to balance well.

To start with, learn how to walk safely and correctly from your Physical Therapist. Your large Achilles tendon in your calf attaches to the foot. You must keep it limber for best balance. If it's tight, it not only hurts and cramps, but it restricts your ability to move your ankle up and down. This is called the "excursion" of the tendon. It is easy to stretch it as an exercise, but it has to be done many times each day to keep it limber. We tighten our muscles and tendons all day long, with the positions in which we sit and move. Because of our bad habits, usually one leg will be tighter than the other. You attend to tightness by stretching. How do you think you attend to one leg being tighter than the other? You guessed it: stretch both legs, but stretch the tighter one a couple of repetitions more than the other.

What you do with your knees, hips, and back also has an effect on your feet and ankles. Take a look; they are all interconnected! Where one goes the rest must follow. Some of the hip and knee muscles connect to the tibia; which is the larger of the two bones in your lower leg. Other hip and knee muscles connect to your pelvis, which, as we discussed earlier, is part of your spine. You know the old song: "the head bone connected to the back bone, the back bone connected to the hip bone…" it's true.

There are many ligaments which criss-cross your ankle to connect the two lower leg bones to each of the seven ankle bones and the nineteen bones in your foot. All these attachments and connections provide you with both the flexibility and stability required for movement. Small muscles in the foot itself also assist in this regard.

The big toe is essential for balance. So much so that it has an inordinate amount of your brain, your Cerebral Motor Cortex, devoted to it. Why? Because it helps you balance and is critically involved with every step you take. It's so important that it has lifting and pushing muscles devoted to it alone. Additionally, it has greater sensory input and feedback capacity so you can use it to your advantage. The minute you think about lifting your big toe, your ankle lifting muscles and those that lift your four smaller toes activate.

Because it has these interconnections and special capacities, it is easiest to think of your big toe with every step while you work on improving your walking pattern. Every time you sit down or rise up, be it a chair, couch, car, or toilet, your big toe is there to help by pushing down on the floor and relaying messages to your brain regarding your movement and stability. Every time you lean back, even just a few degrees, your big toe and ankle muscles quickly activate to help your abdominal and hip muscles to bring you forward, and back into balance. When you lean forward; your big toe signals your brain which in turn signals your calf, hip, and back muscles to help them bring you upright again. When it occurs side to side these same inputs and muscles activate to center you.

Circling your ankles and wiggling your toes while you are sitting is a way to increase flexibility, circulation, and gain some strength; however, it's not enough. The greatest aid to your balance is to be upright, on your feet and ankles. You'll get the maximum in strength, sensory input, and feedback. Practicing what you've been exposed to, reminded by, and taught in this book is the imperative for the improvement of your balance and the ongoing improvement in your life.

However, if you sit much of the day and rarely move; your response times slow, muscles weaken, joints, ligaments, tendons, and muscles start to stiffen. Your balance is impaired. It's a threat to your lifestyle, and maybe your life.

Every part of you depends on all the other parts of you. The nice thing is when you practice the ideas in this book you'll find the ideas are repeated in several different ways; but they are all the same basic ideas. Therefore, you only have to remember a few basic concepts. Each is something you learned earlier in your life, and as such your brain will respond quickly, when and if you care to re-teach the lessons. You were born to move often and in balance.

Chapter Five

"Bits and Pieces"

I want to close by encouraging you. Working on you balance is well worth the effort. No one can guarantee that you won't fall. I've watched hundreds of people in our small town work faithfully on their balance. They are so thankful for having made the effort and for the positive changes, big and small. They often say that they better understand how their body works, what it needs, and how to evaluate their walking and other daily activities with respect to their balance habits. Many have special circumstances: arthritis, diabetes, Parkinson's disease, M.S., and strokes. Some use walkers and canes, but they use them more to their advantage now. They wear supportive shoes, added more night lights, threw out those "sloppy slippers", and move to music when they can.

I've been enthusiastically encouraging throughout this work, but I don't want to offer false hope. We can't regain all the natural balance of our early youth, and no amount of re-teaching will fully repair that which is irreparably damaged. However, that said, you'll never know what's possible if you don't try. Your decision, your commitment, and your perseverance are the first second and third hurdles that only you can approach and surmount. Be thoughtful and logical but enjoy yourself. Feel your new energy building and realize that in many ways you are in control of your health, your brain, and your body. You get to choose.

I want you to be informed and empowered. I want you to understand how your body works. I want to open your eyes to the opportunities that surround you every day. I want you to see that, done properly what you do will make a difference. I want you to be the best person you can, and enjoy a healthy life on your way forward.

Improve your balance and improve your life; it's your choice.